Scrap The Book - Read A Cartoon

Also by Donna Daugherty

On The Sine
Growing Up
Where The Wind Blows
It's About Cooking and Caring For Family
Hug Me While You Can
Childhood Folk Tales and Stories
The Dawtree Clinic: Amyloidosis
How to Be A Sucessful Travel Nurse
Gift Poem For Nurses
Scrap The Book - Read A Cartoon
Sissy and Her Cat: Scratch
Biblical Answers To Everyday Problems
David Goes Down Under
David and The Knobby Knot Hole
Andrew Goes To Homeschool
Run! It's A Decoy
Adult Coloring Book Women
Adult Coloring Book Sea Monster Cartoons

Donna Daugherty, RN

Scrap The Book - Read A Cartoon

Scrap The Book - Read A Cartoon

Copyright © 2018, 2013 Donna Daugherty, RN
All Rights Reserved.

ISBN: 9781731000422 (paperback edition)
ASIN: B00CHFQ212 (ebook edition)

This book or parts thereof may not be reproduced in any form by any means – electronic, mechanical, photocopy, recording or otherwise – without prior written permission of the publisher, except as provided by the United States of America copyright law.

Neither the author nor the publisher take any responsibility for the loss to any person or organization acting or refraining from action as a result of information obtained from this publication.

Characters in this book are fictitious. Any similarity to real persons, living or dead, is coincidental and not intended by the author.

Graphics
Nurse Hazel from the cartoon, *Scrap The Book - Read A Cartoon*
By Donna Daugherty (Donet')

PRINTED IN THE UNITED STATES OF AMERICA

Scrap The Book - Read A Cartoon

Make every day count with Nurse Hazel's 'Scrap the Book - Read A Cartoon'.

She's so serious that she's just hilarious! She's read all of the policies and procedures; just trying to follow the ever changing rules and regulations of the health care reform.

She's shocked from the time she gets to work until the time she leaves. She can't seem to find that one compliant patient.

... Nurse Hazel Products ...
BUY Nurse Hazel Cartoon T-Shirts, Mugs, Aprons, Mousepads, Bags and more.

http://www.HappyFishGallery.com

Nurse Hazel, your favorite cartoon nurse, and the comic world of medicine.

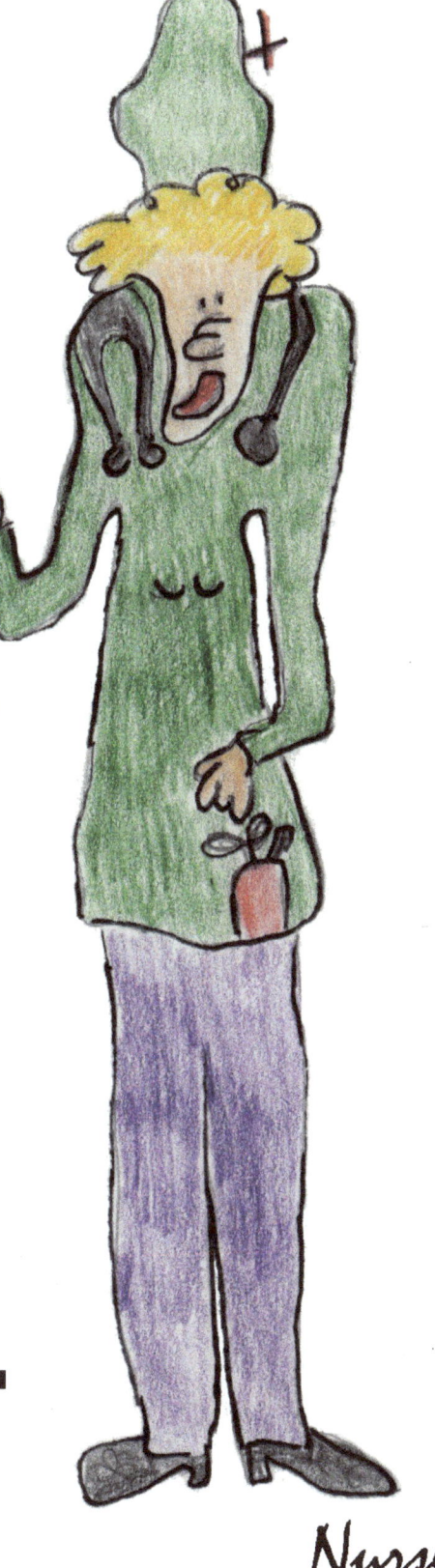

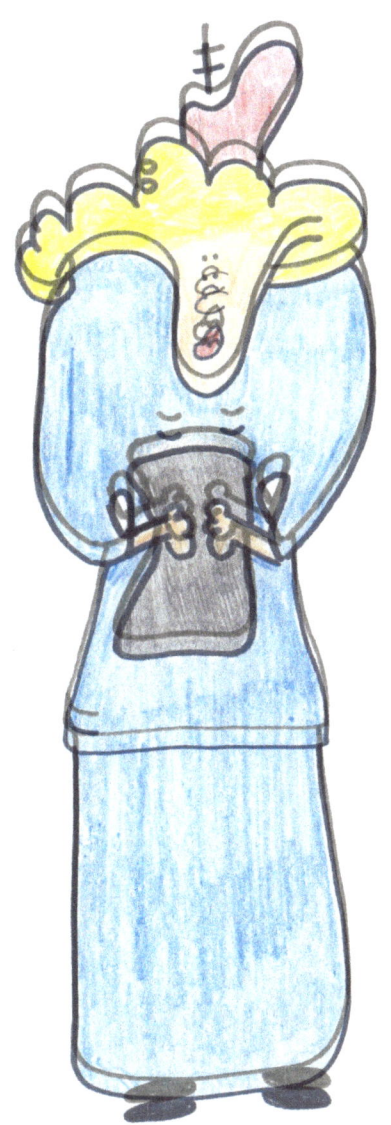

One nurse blew out her knee,
the other called in blowing it
out both ends. If this keeps up,
we'll have to bring in blow up nurses.
All we need now
is a nurse to come in blowing fumes.

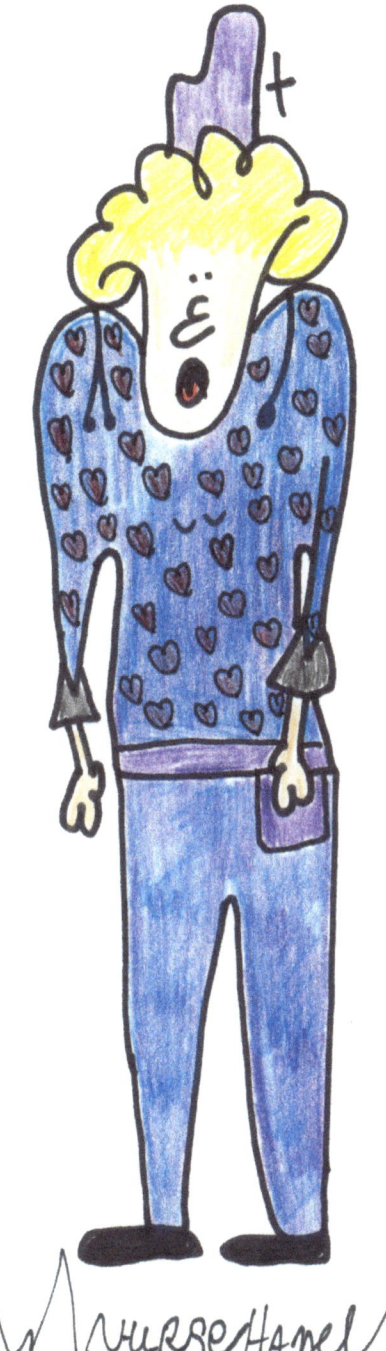

Can you just email me the rest of this report!

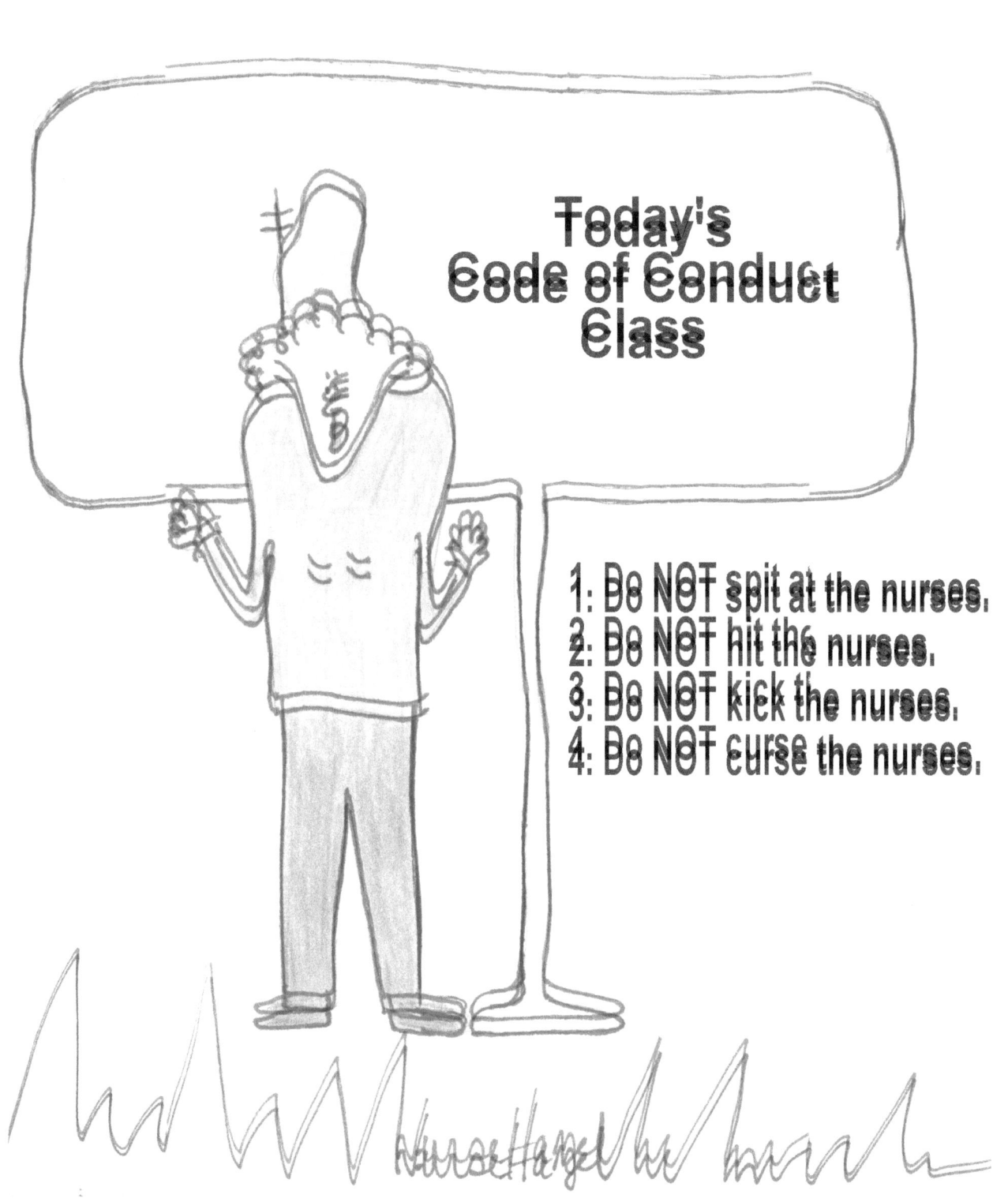

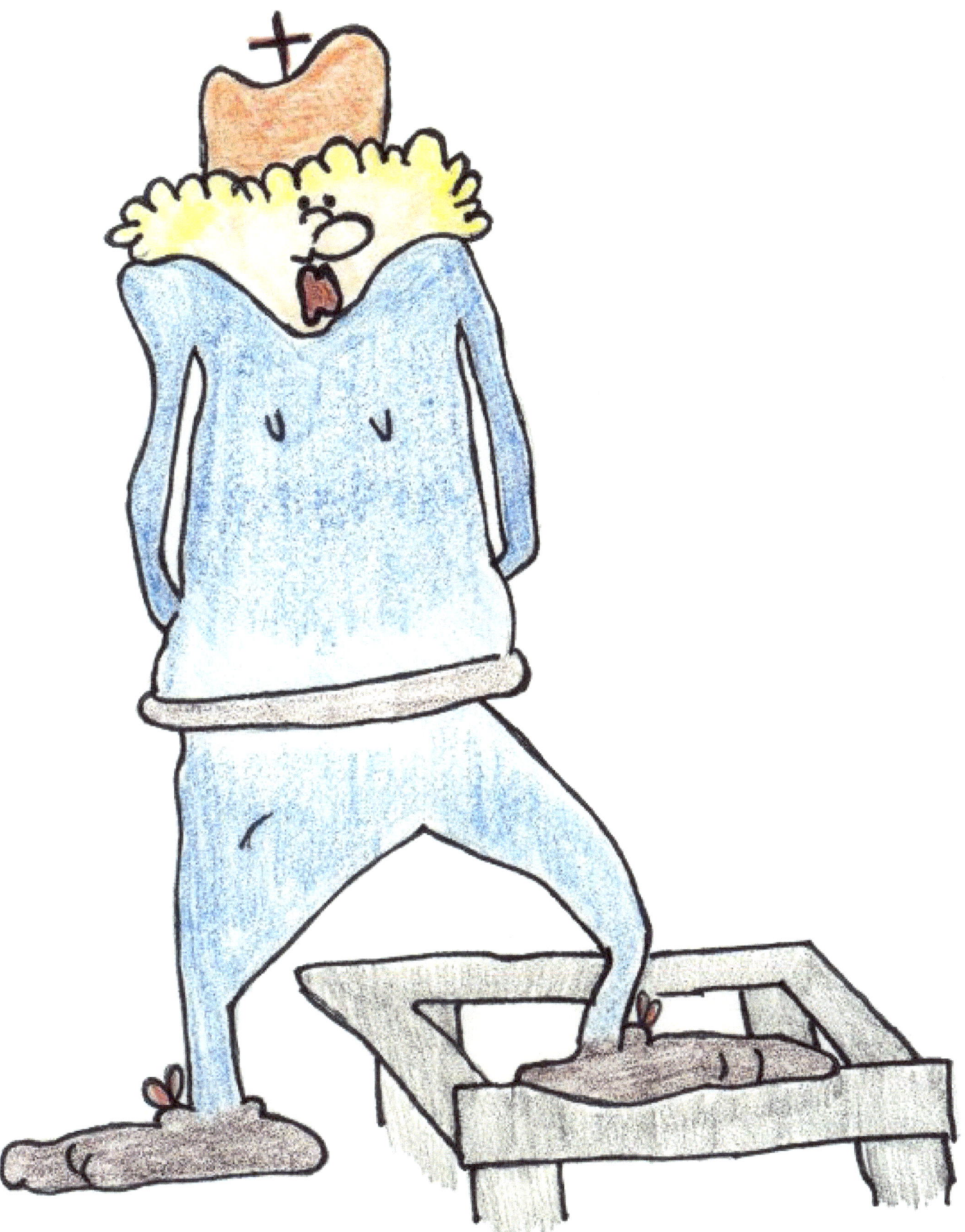

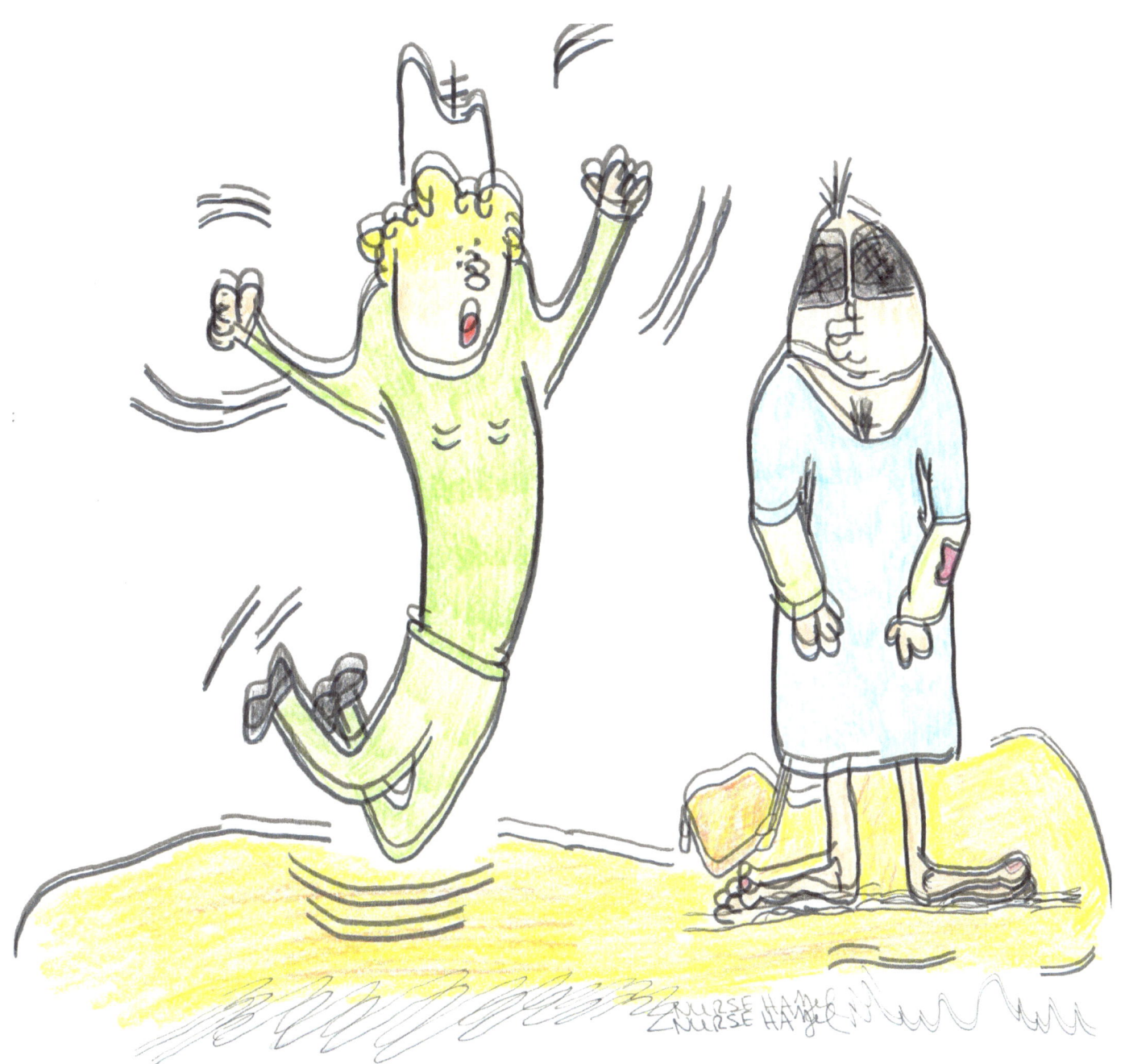

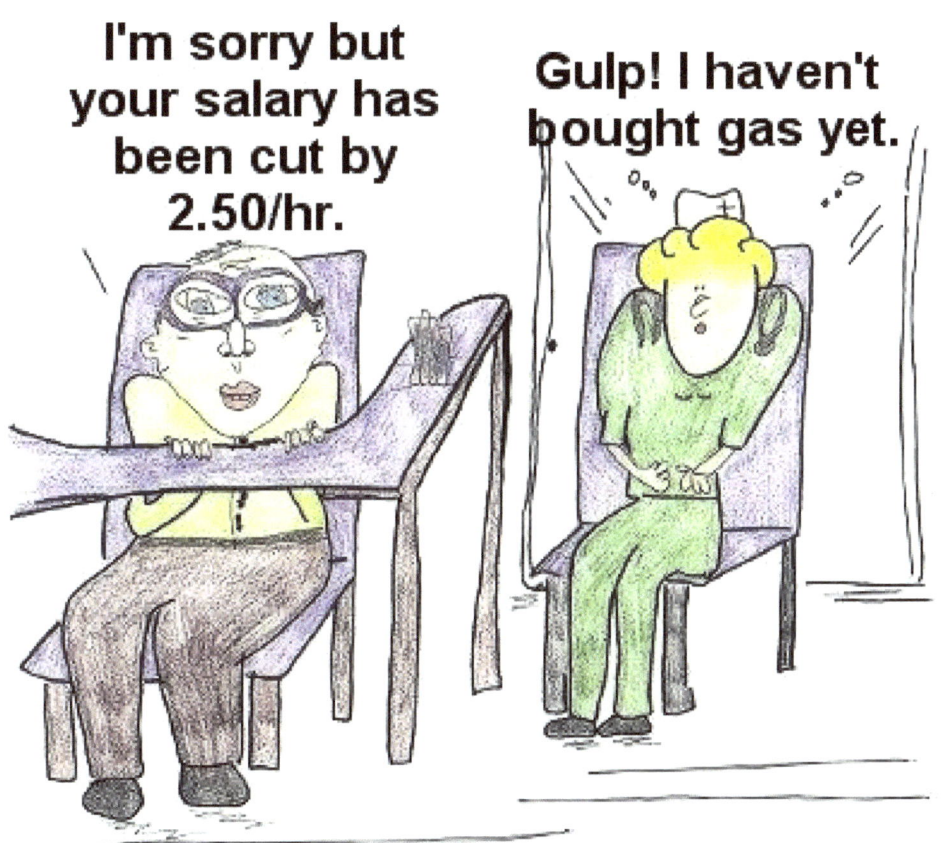

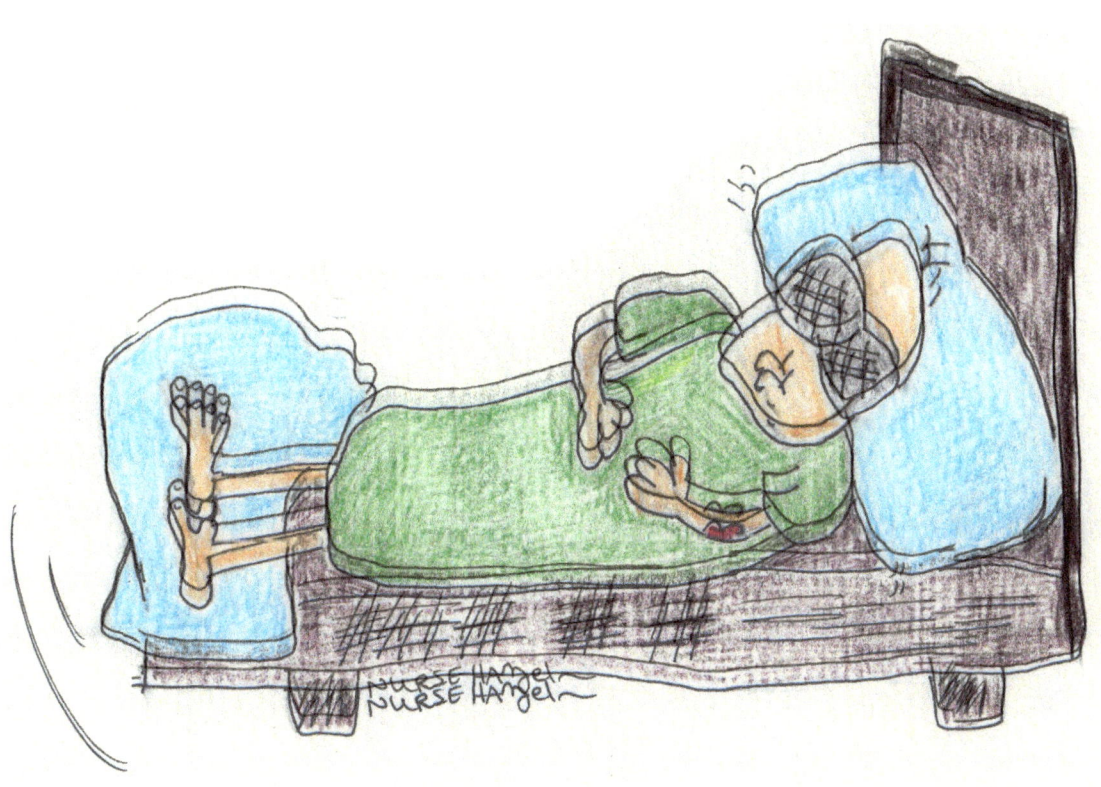

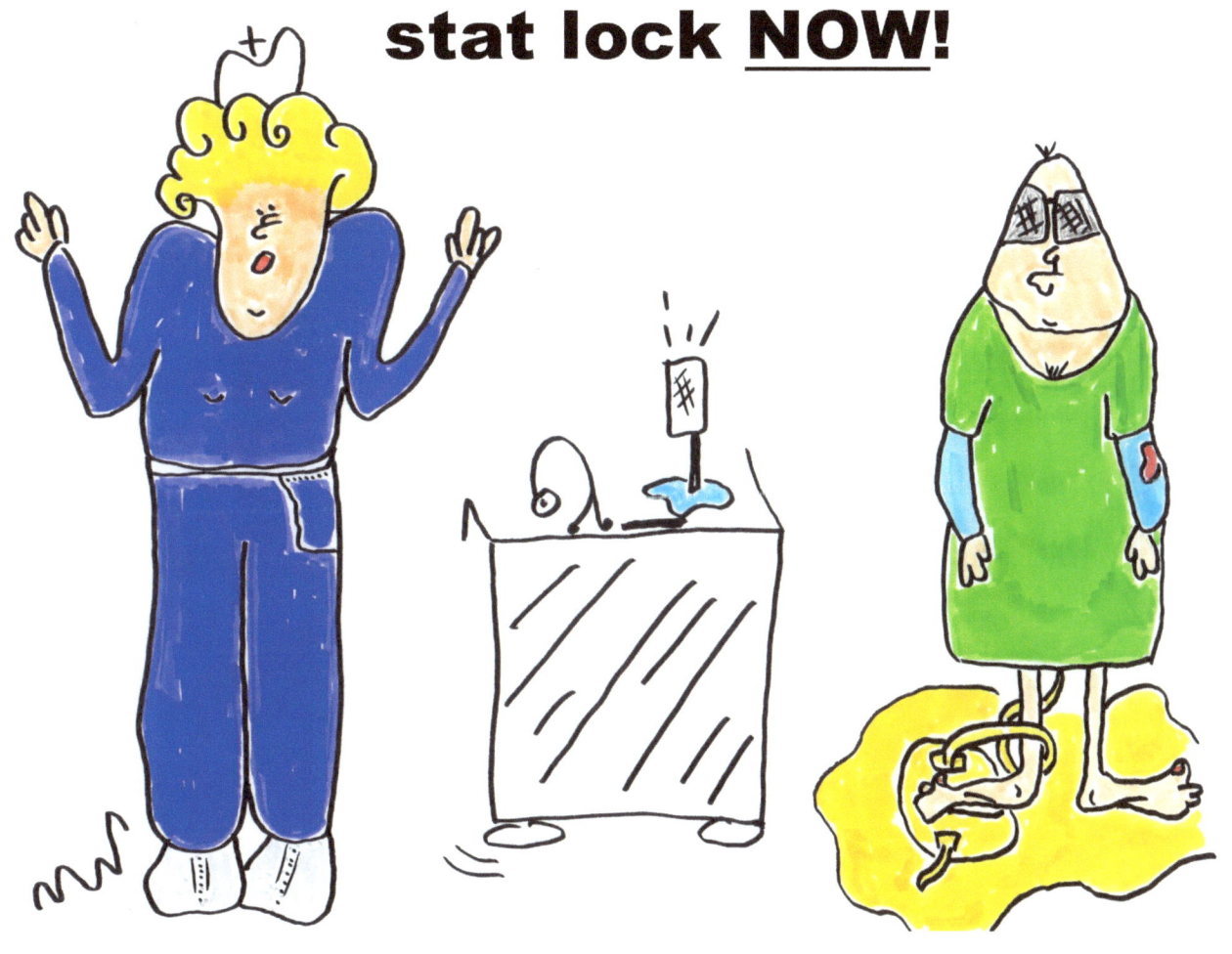

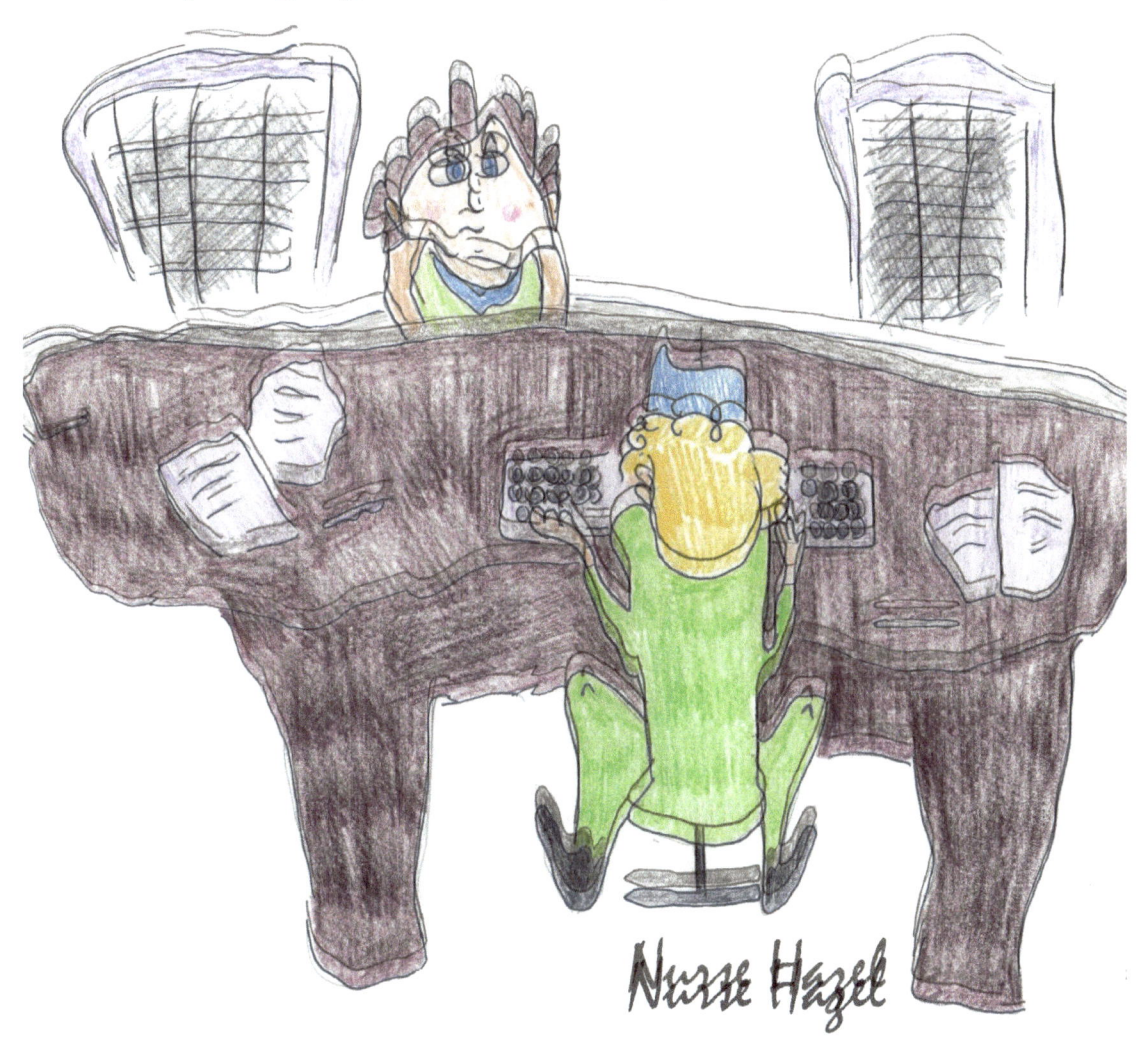

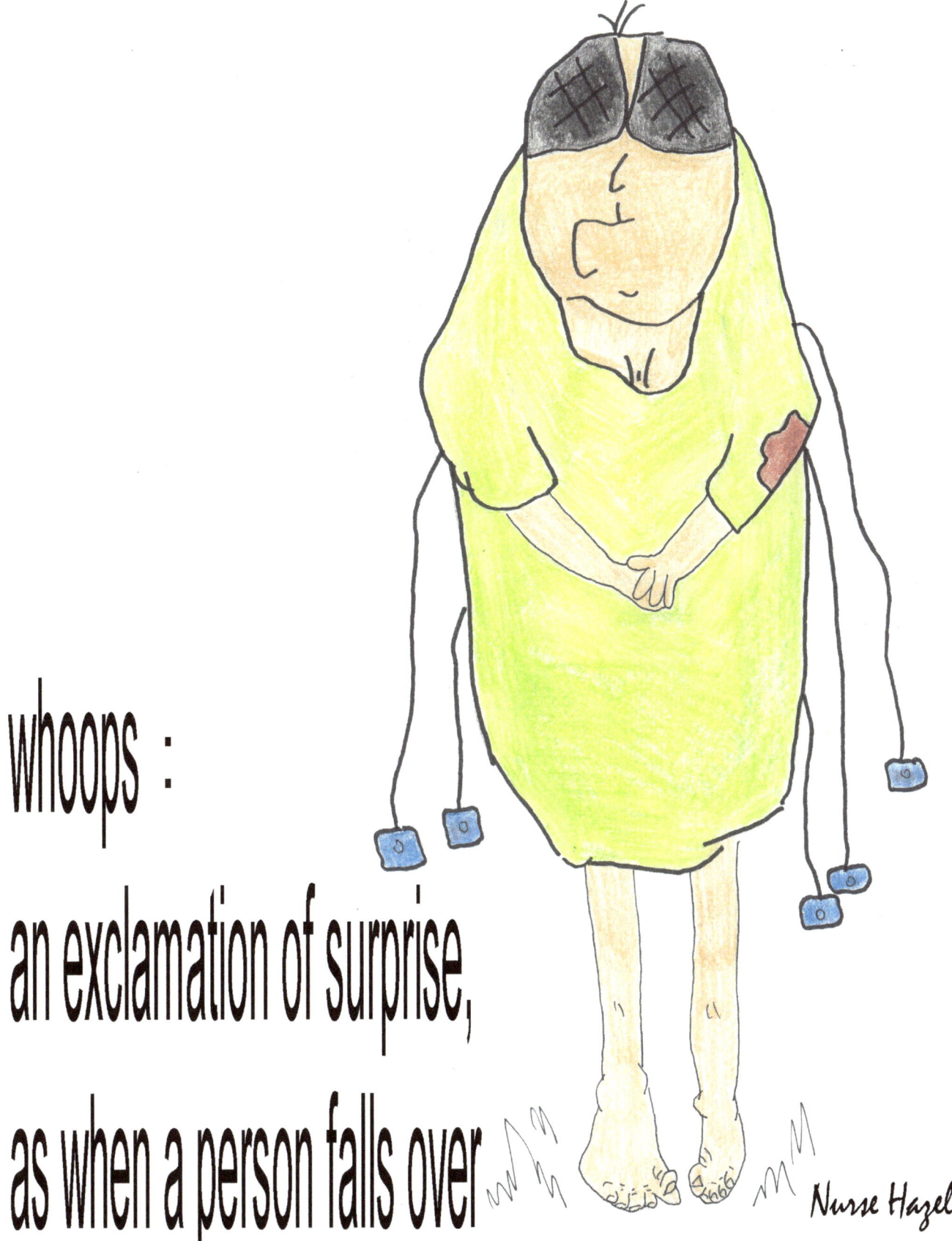

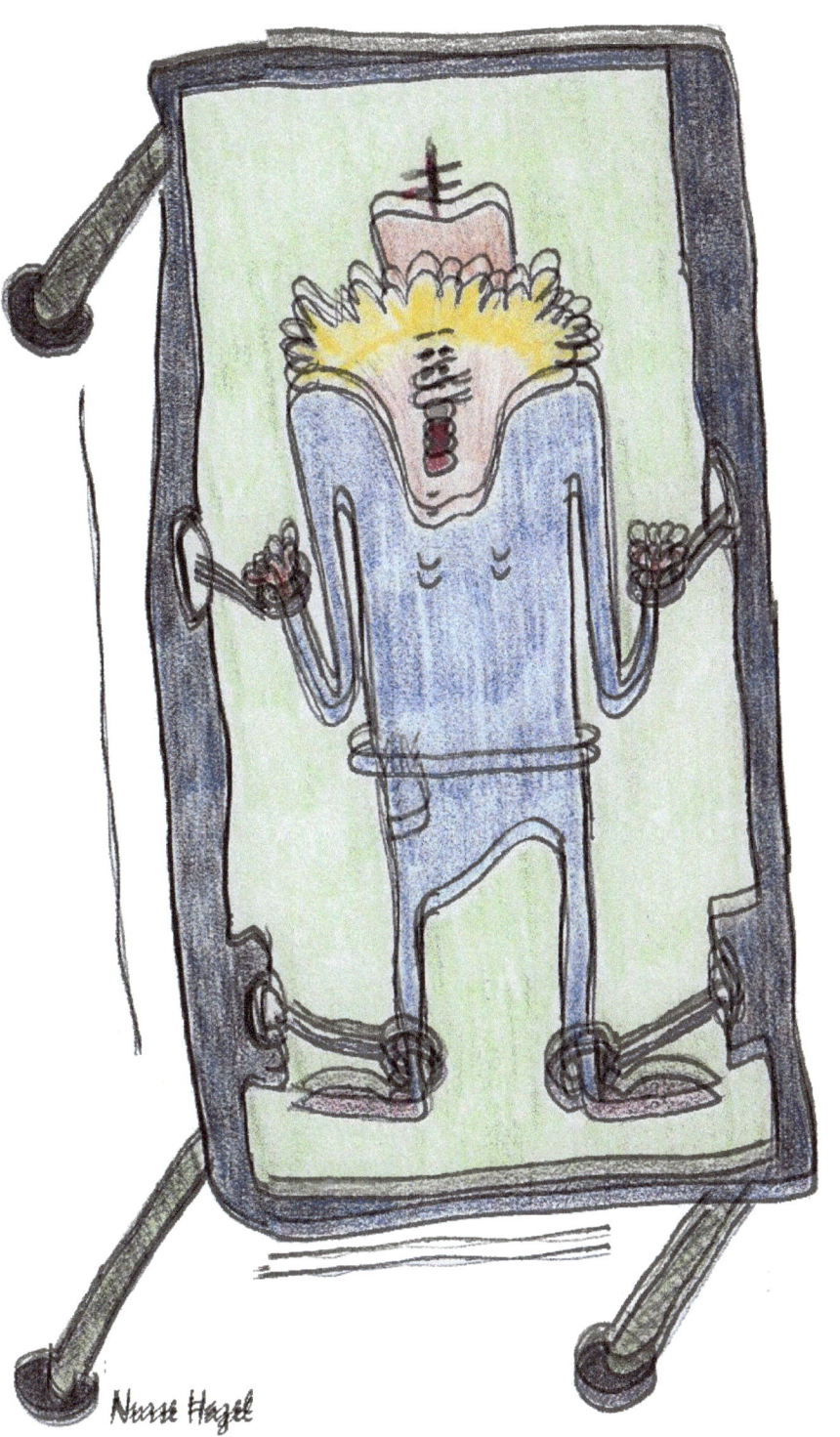

Do I have to buy you another going away cake?

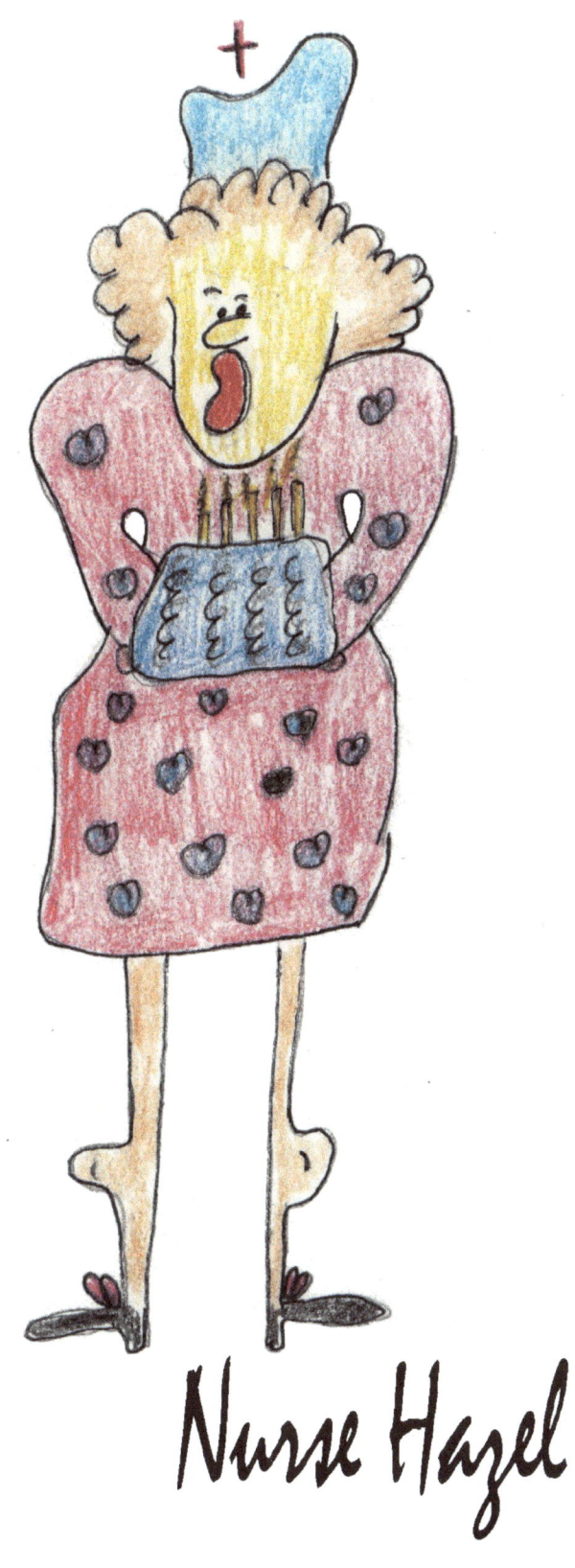

Nurse Hazel

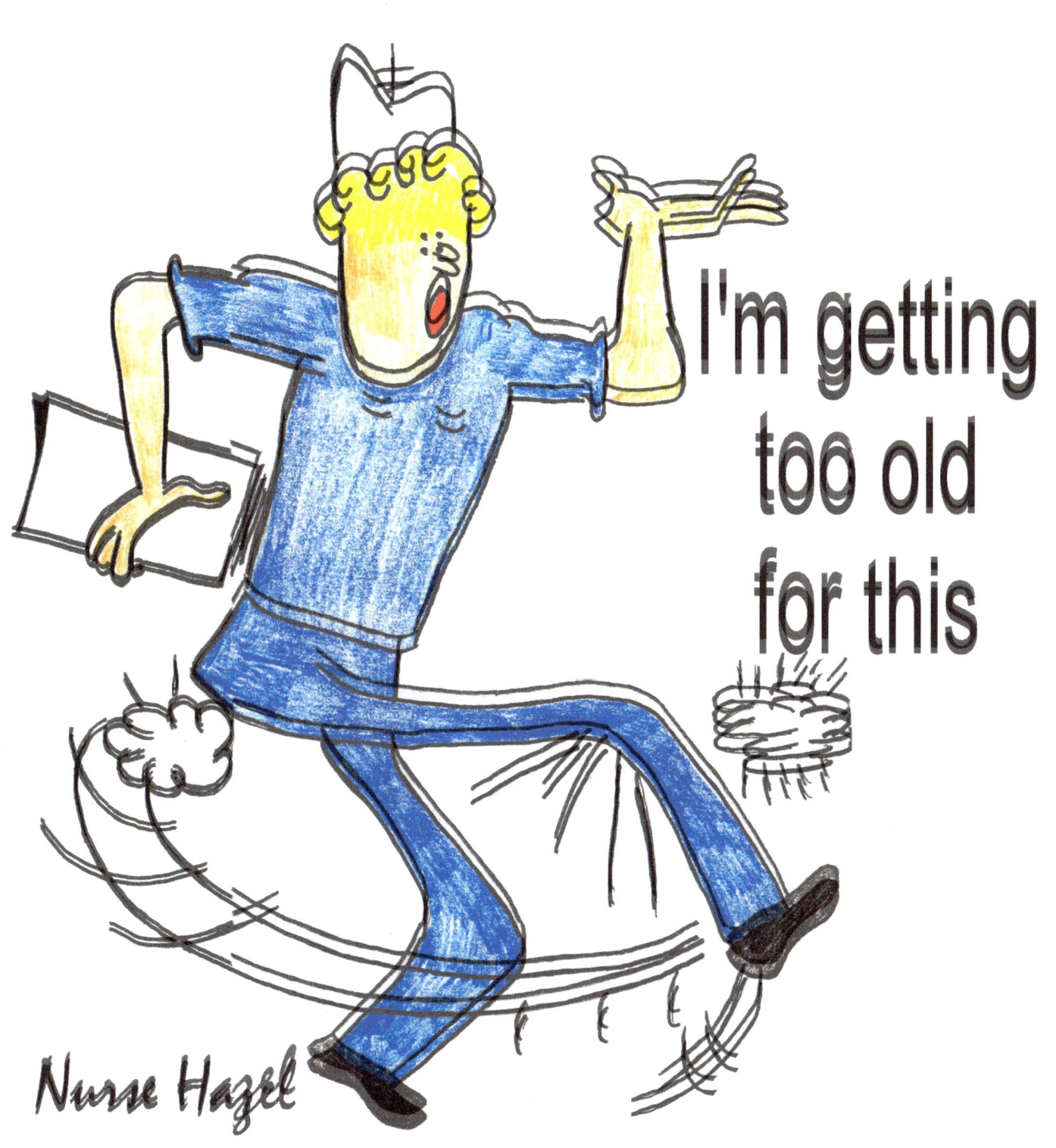

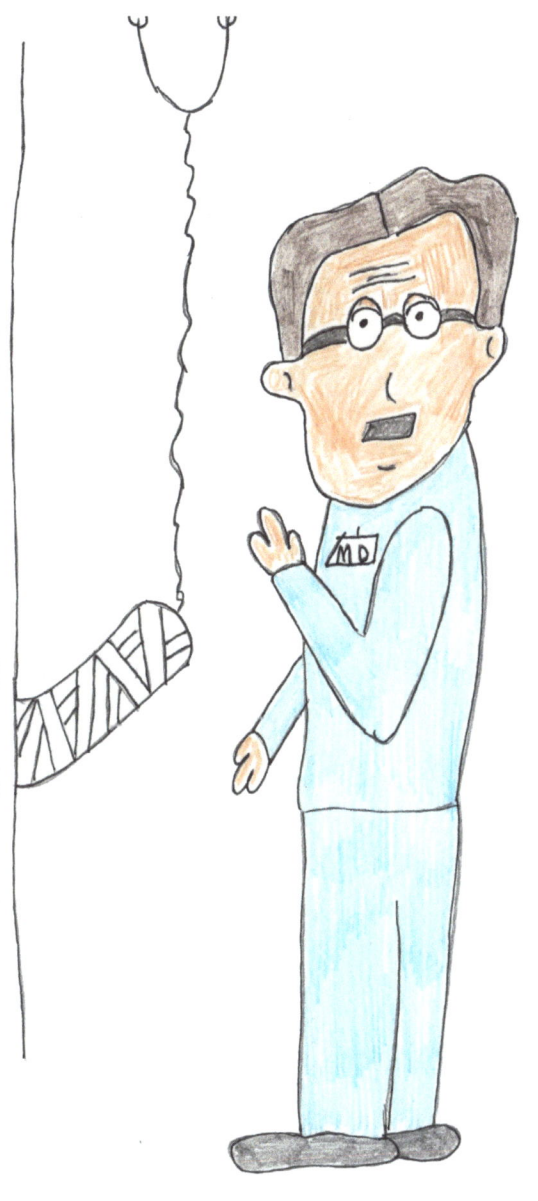

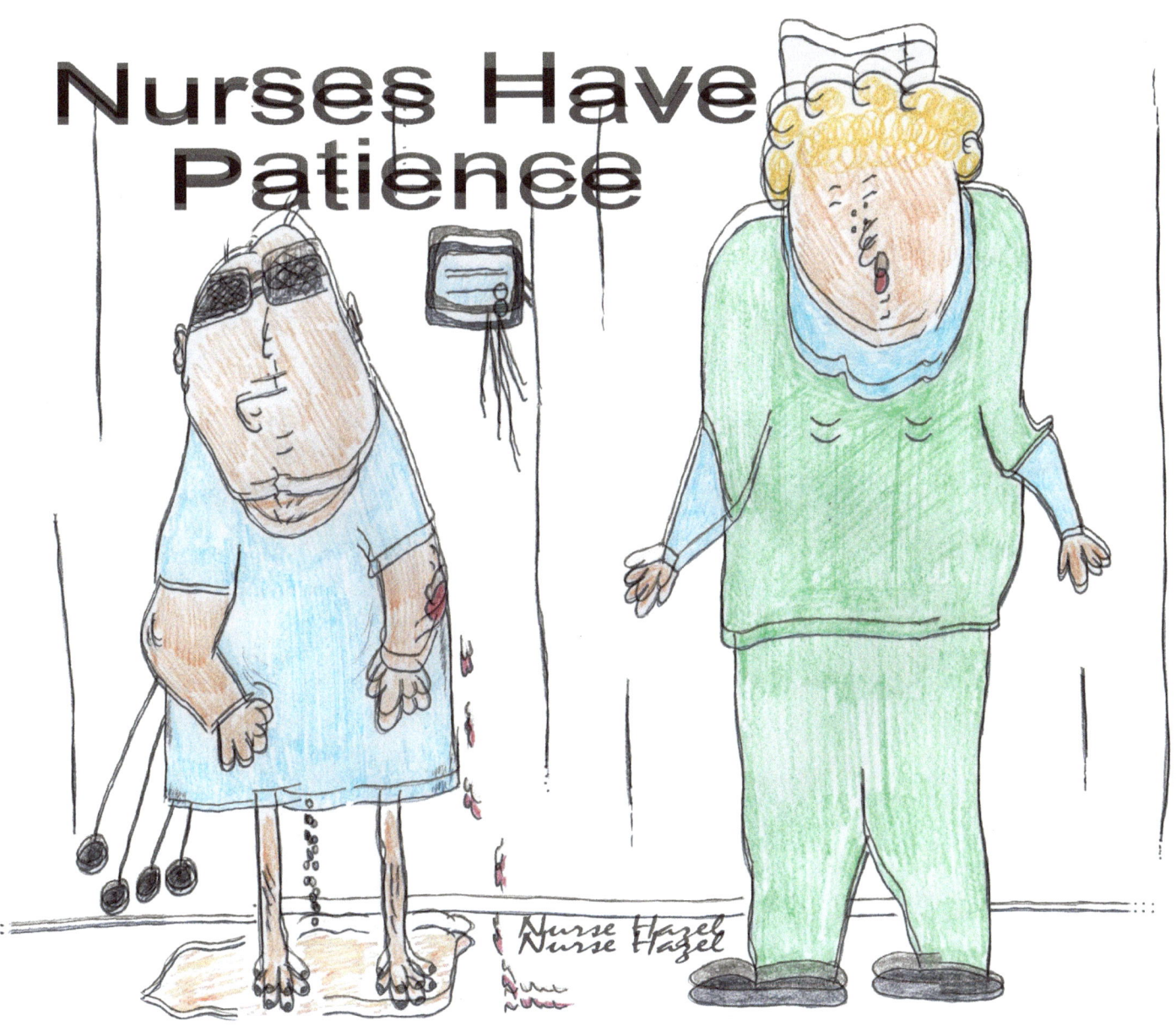

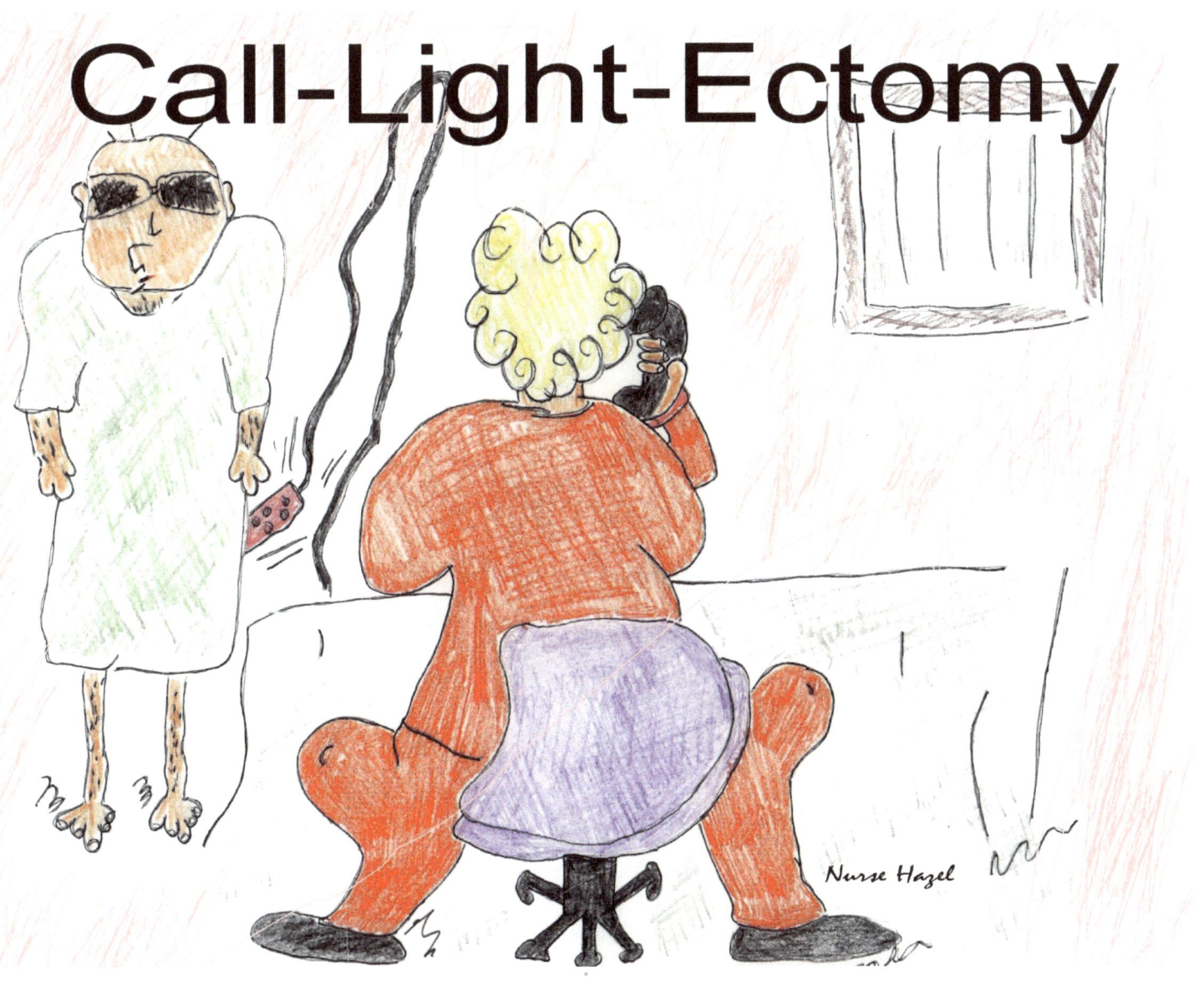

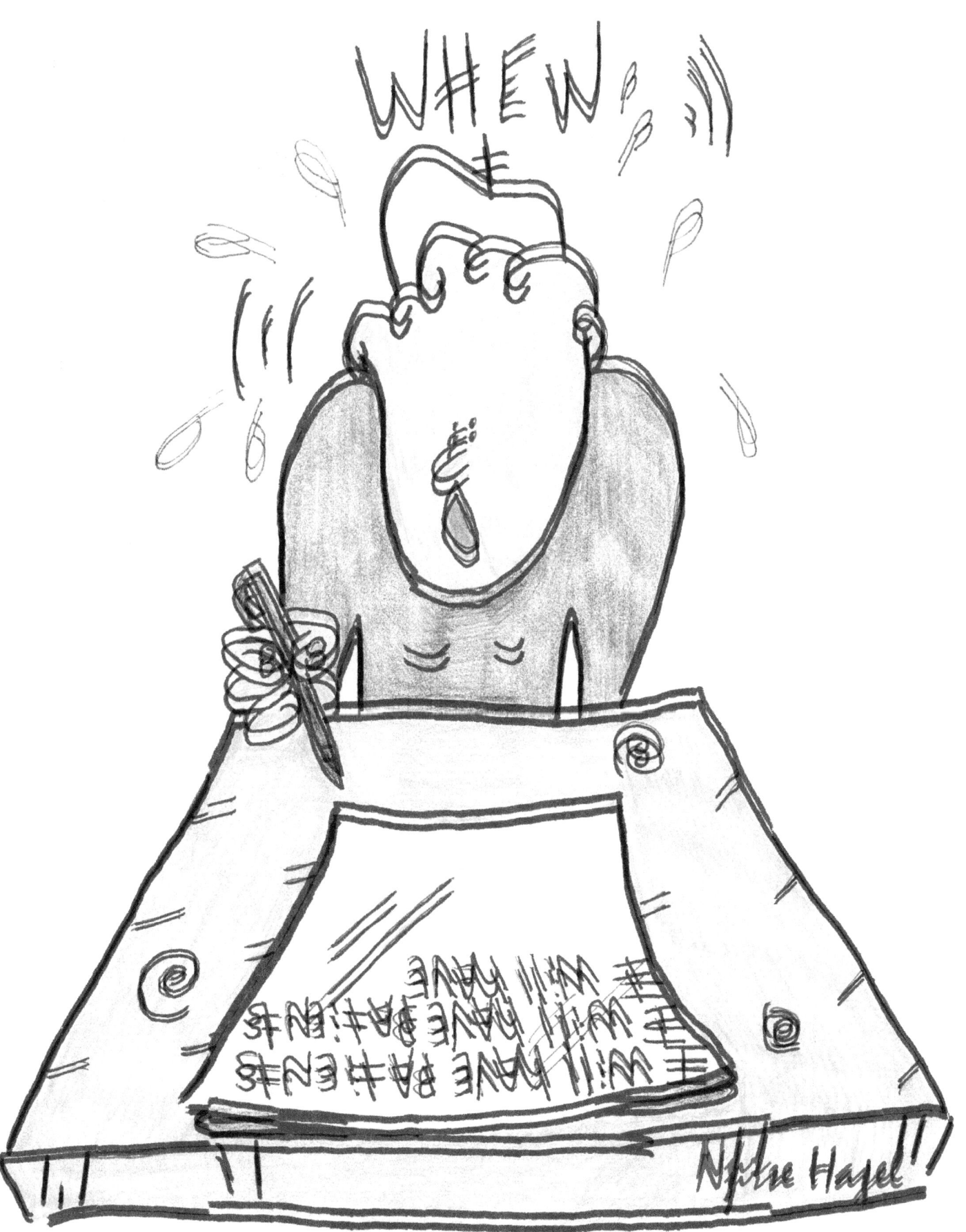

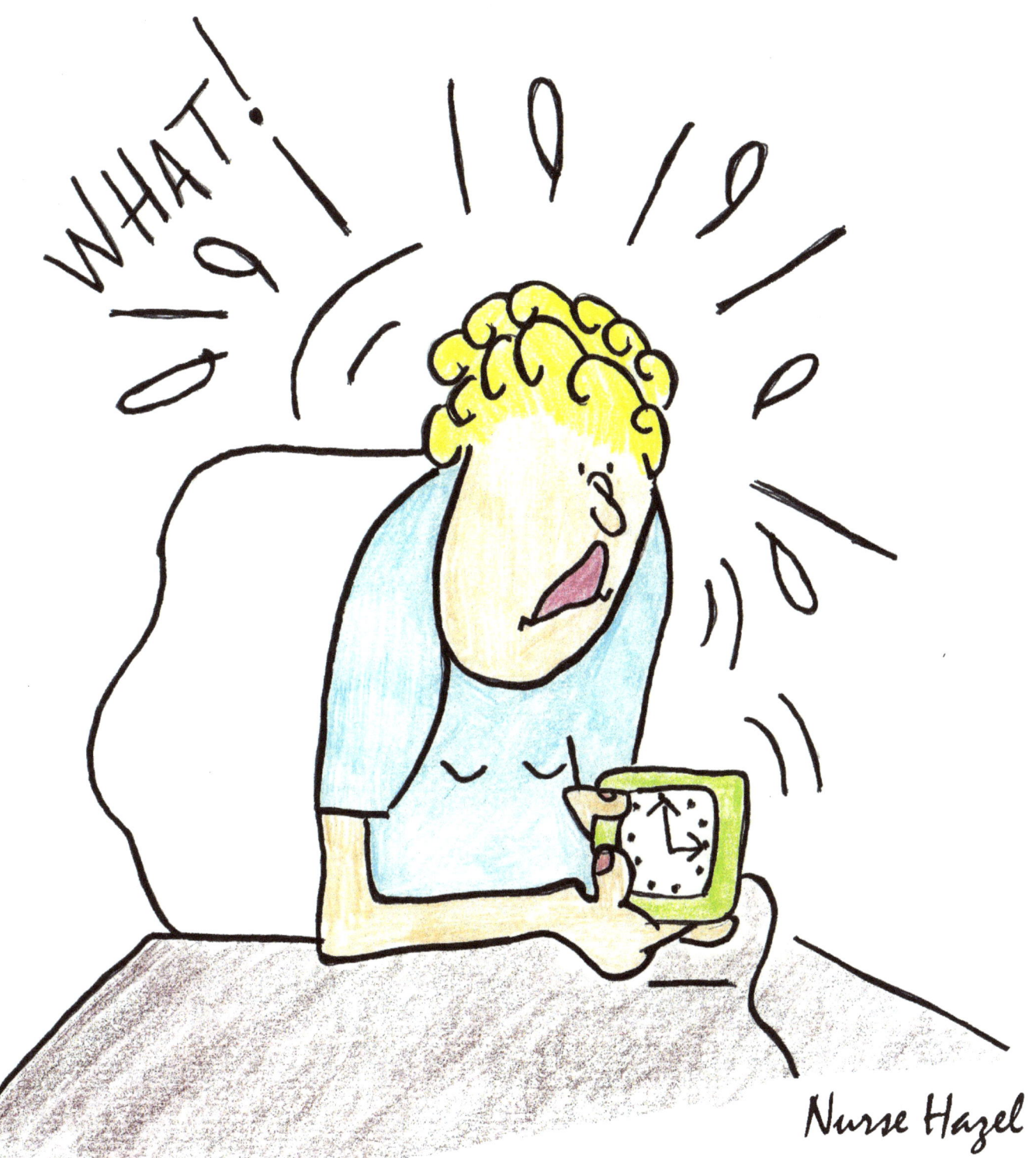

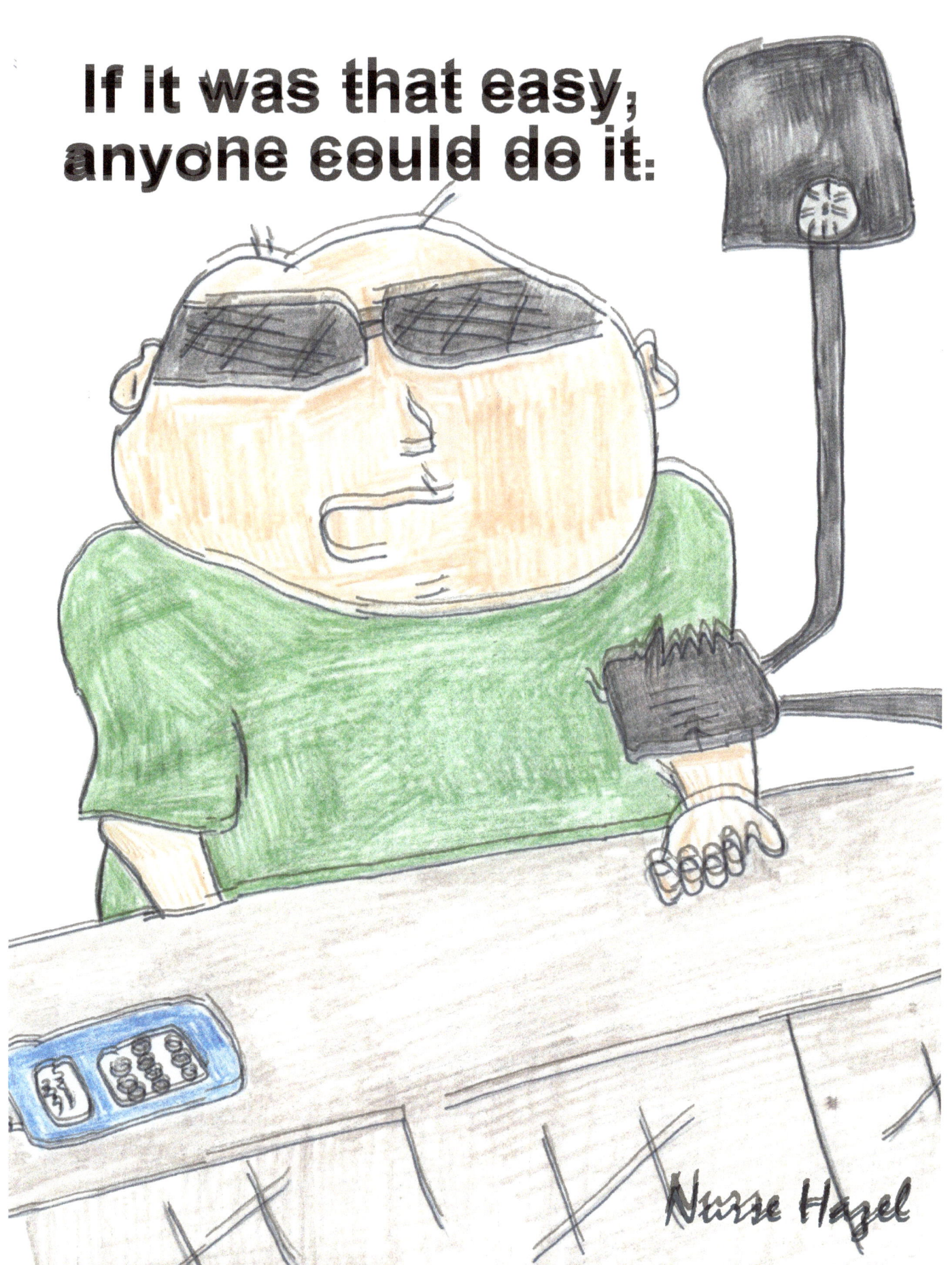

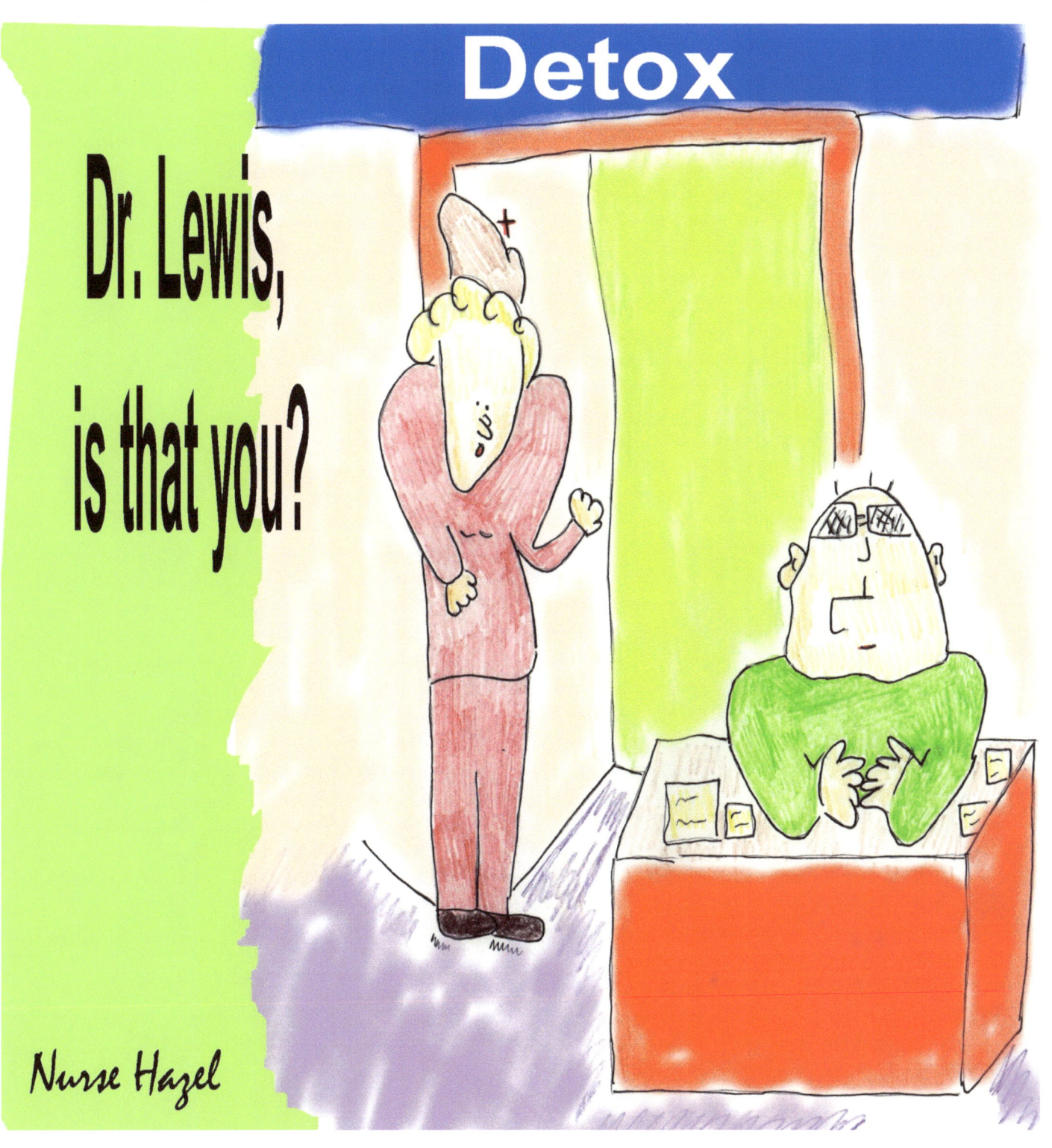

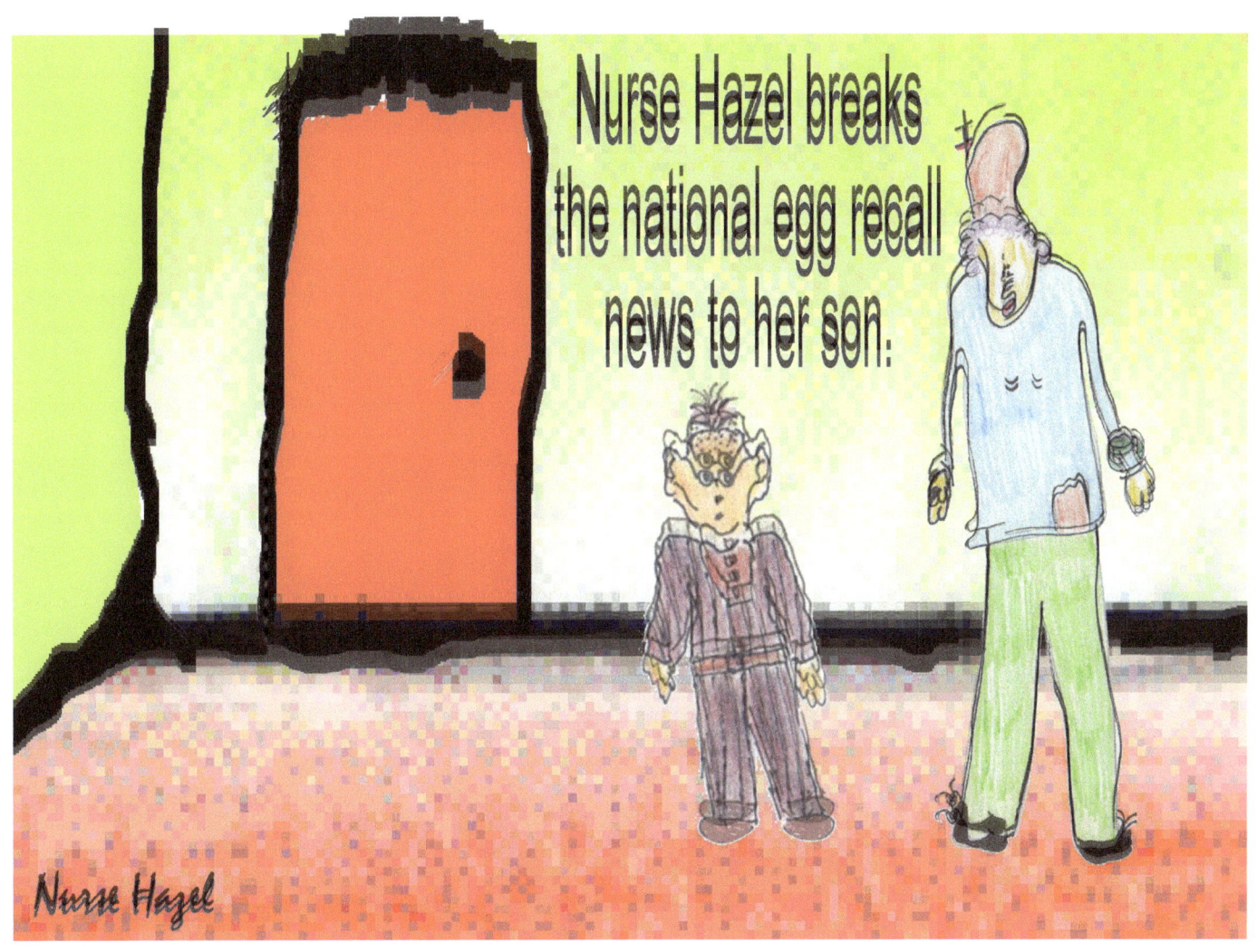

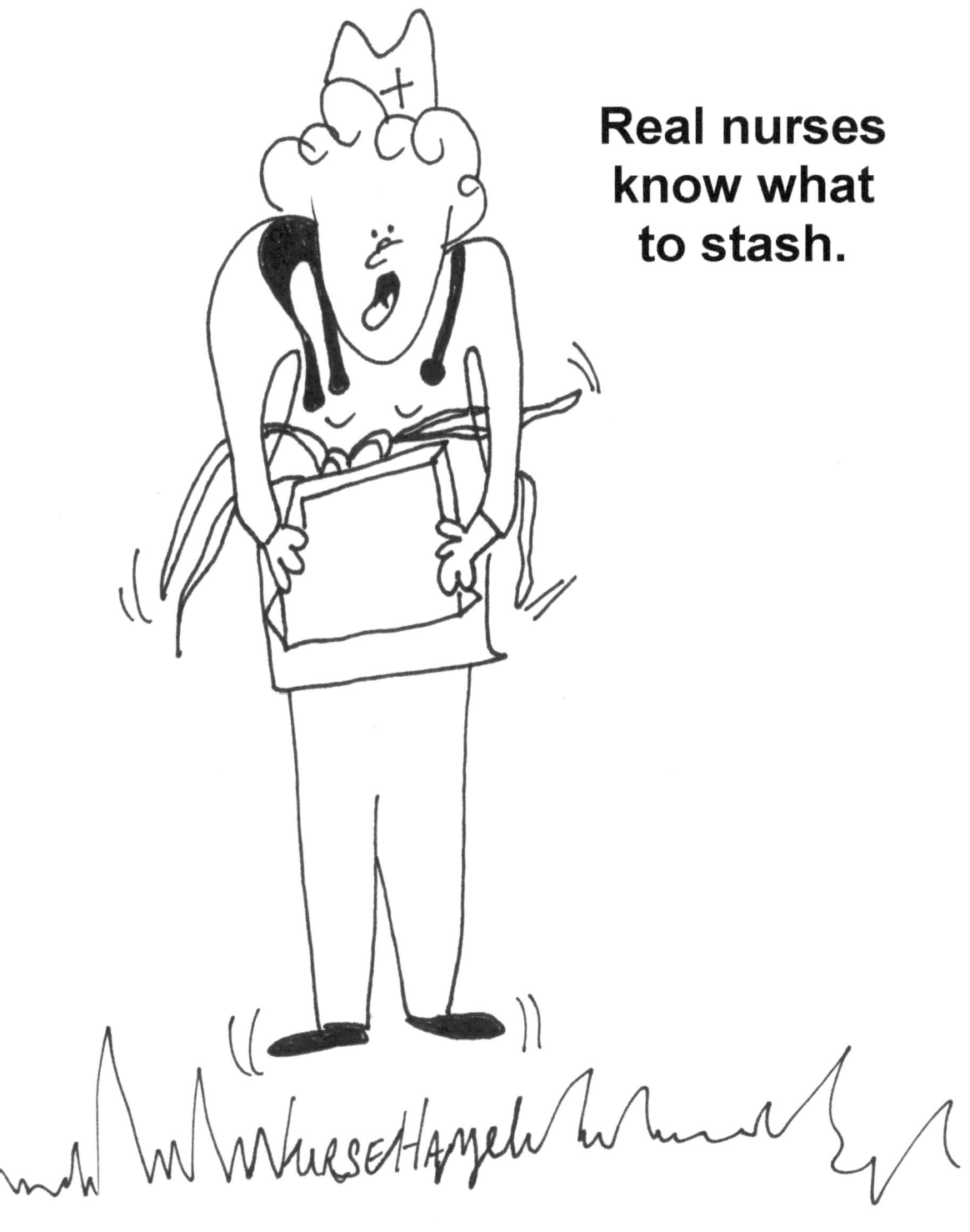

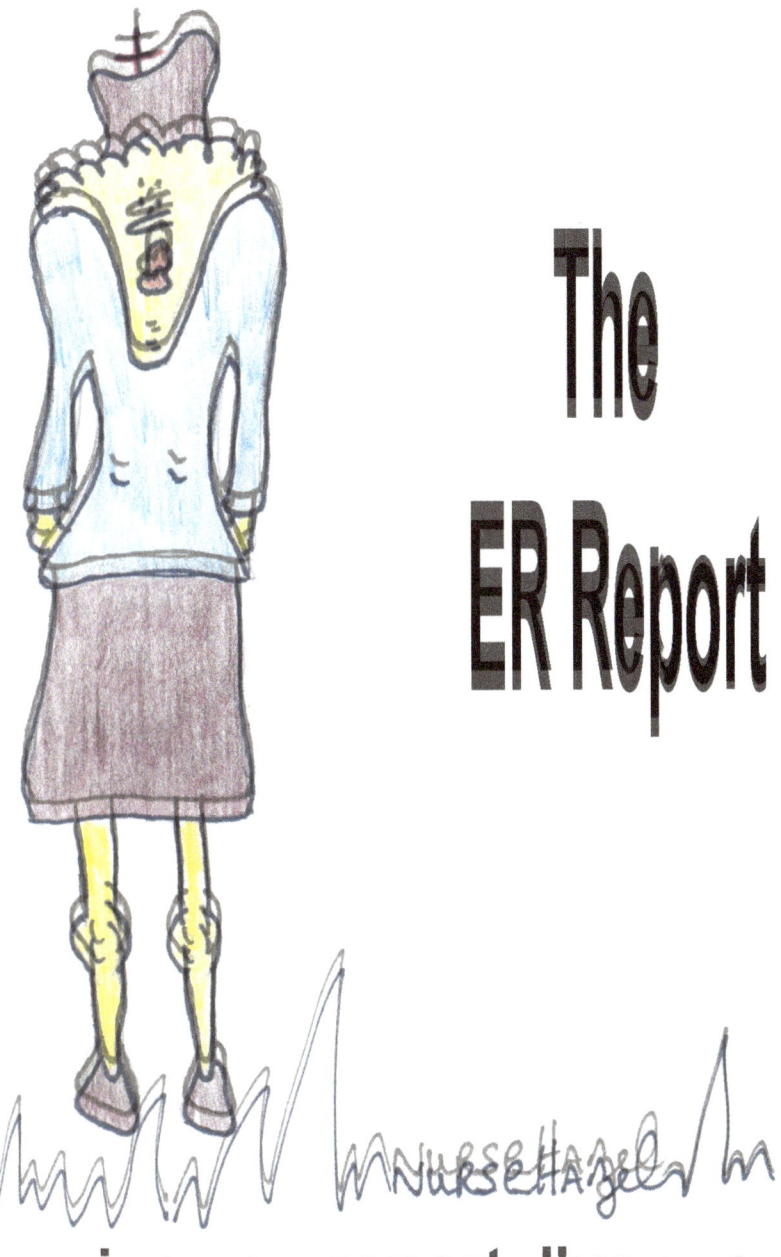

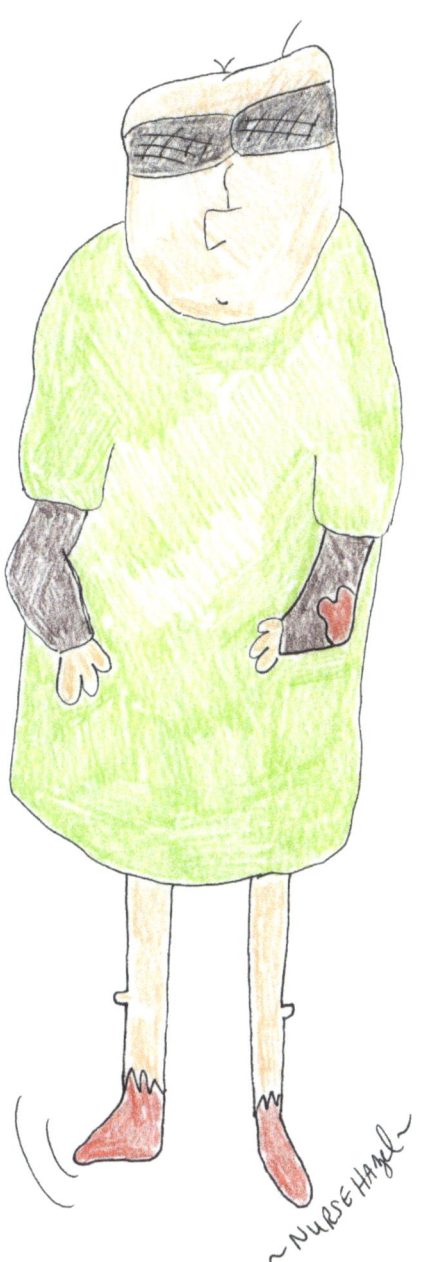

Nurses Pain Scale

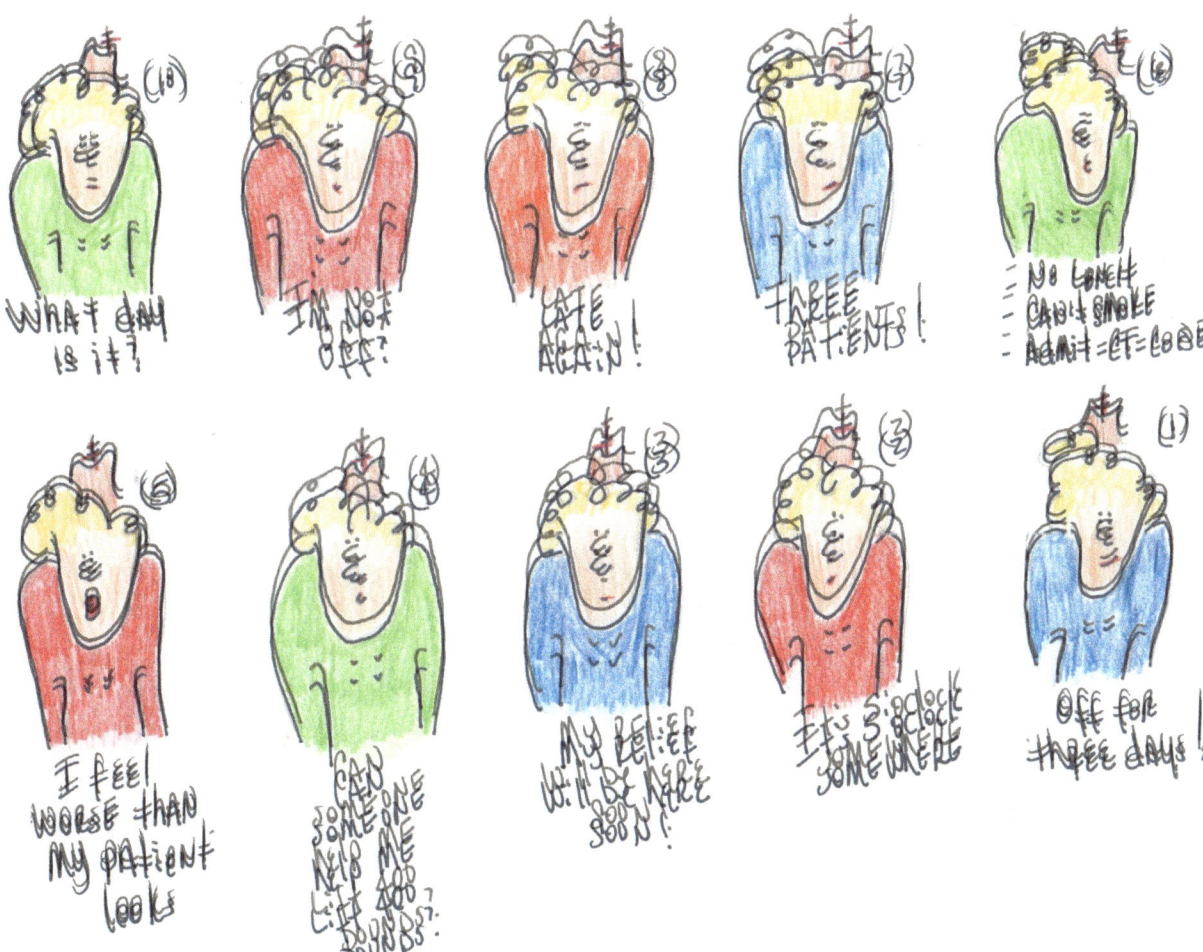

About The Author

Donna Daugherty is an American born, freelance writer and graphics designer. She enjoys working as an ICU critical care nurse. Walking on the beach with her husband and dog (Eor), and talking about the characters in her books, are favorite hobbies.

She's been a writer most of her life, from poems to songs to short stories. A favorite daydream is writing a biography that includes the statement, "Her latest book has won the Pulitzer Prize".

Genres: Science Fiction, Fiction, Children's Stories and Songs, All Occasion Poems, Nurse Hazel Cartoons, Sissy and Her Cat Scratch Cartoons, Christian Books and Songs.

Please visit our publisher at PWPMall.com for other products that we carry.

Many products available with the characters included in this book.

www.ingramcontent.com/pod-product-compliance
Lightning Source LLC
Chambersburg PA
CBHW051919210526
45473CB00006B/2072